THE DISCOVERY OF HEALTH –PROGRAMMING LANGUAGE

LANGUAGE

BY

RAHALI LAWALI

TABLE OF CONTENTS   Page No.

INTRODUCTION

The **health** of each and every individual is at risk of contacting one kind of an **infection**, **disease** or **tumor** at one of the three – transitional stages of human development, namely: pre, intra and post delivery. Hence, if the final outcome of the contact is in favor of infection, disease or tumor, it is the **death** that would be celebrating, but if the final outcome of the contact is in favor of **treatment**, the patient [**life**] and various heath personnel would be jubilating, and they include **doctors, nurses, radiologists, scientists** and **pharmacists** contributing at various capacities. In this scenario the cardinal features of a modern health settlement has been depicted. There is a programming language in support of this scenario which will be communicated to the readers shortly.

HEALTH- PROGRAMMING LANGUAGE

It is important to note that what we know about health is basically designed using a programming language that has three main components, namely:

-*Health- Segmented Code*
-*Health -Integrated Code*
- *Health-Organ Of Interest*

1-HEALTH- SEGMENTED CODE

Working From The First Dimension, We Have:

Input= [O^I x Q] A Slide per Letter

INPUT = HEALTH

DATA

O -26

I - 6letters: 5, 4,3,2,1,0

Q-h= 7, e =4, a = 0, l = 11, t=19, h= 7

COMPUTING

h[26^5 x 7] + e[26^4 x 4] +a [26^3 x 0] +l[26^2 x 11] + t[26^1 x 19] + h[26^0 x 7]

OUTPUT IN FIGURES

[85005473]-this is the Cardinal value of the word 'health'

Hence, to derive *Health-Segmented Code*, each one of the definite digit inside the above cardinal values need to appear only once.

[85005473]= **[8-5-4-7-3]**-Health-Segmented Code

Interpretation Of Heath-Segmented Code

 INPUT = HOSPITAL

COMPUTING

 h[26^7 x 7] + o[26^6 x 14] +s[26^5 x 18] + p[26^4 x 15] +i[26^3 x 8]

+t[26^2 x 19] + a[26^1 x 0] + l[26^0 x 11]

OUTPUT

[60768364967]

[53]

[**8**]-[**8**-5-4-7-3]

It implies that hospital is among the right places to go for making health inquiries.

INPUT = CHEMIST

COMPUTING

 c[26^6 x 2] +h[26^5 x 7] + e[26^4 x 4] +m[26^3 x 12] +i[26^2 x 8] + s[26^1 x 18] + t[26^0 x 19]

OUTPUT

[703045895]

[41]

[**5**]-[8-**5**-4-7-3]

It implies that chemist is among the right places to go for making health inquiries.

INPUT = HEALTH CLINIC

COMPUTING

h[26^5 x 7] + e[26^4 x 4] +a [26^3 x 0] +l[26^2 x 11] + t[26^1 x 19] + h[26^0 x 7]/+/ c[26^5 x 2] + l[26^4 x 11] +i[26^3 x 8] +n[26^2 x 13] + i[26^1 x 8] + c[26^0 x 2]

OUTPUT

[703045895]+[28939094]

[731984989]

[58]

[13]

[4]-[8-5-4-7-3]

It implies that health clinic is among the right places to go for making health inquiries.

INPUT = MEDICAL STORE

COMPUTING

m[26^6 x 12] +e[26^5 x 4] + d[26^4 x 3] +i [26^3 x 8] +c[26^2 x 2] + a[26^1 x 0] + l[26^0 x 11] /+/ s[26^4 x 18] +t[26^3 x 19] +o[26^2 x 14] + r[26^1 x 17] + e[26^0 x 4]

OUTPUT

[3756027715   ]+[8569422]

[3764597137]

[52]

[7]-[8-5-4-7-3]

It implies that medical store is among the right places to go for making health inquiries

INPUT = PRIMARY HEALTHCARE CENTER

COMPUTING

$p[26^6$ x 15] +r$[26^5$ x 17] + i$[26^4$ x 8] + m$[26^3$ x 12] +a$[26^2$ x 0] + r$[26^1$ x 17] + y$[26^0$ x 24] /+/ h$[26^9$ x 7] + e$[26^8$ x 4] + a$[26^7$ x 0] + l$[26^6$ x 11] +t$[26^5$ x 19] + h$[26^4$ x 7] +c$[26^3$ x 2] +a$[26^2$ x 0] + r$[26^1$ x 17] + e$[26^0$ x 4]/+/ +c$[26^5$ x 2] + e$[26^4$ x 4] +n$[26^3$ x 13] +t$[26^2$ x 19] + e$[26^1$ x 4] + r$[26^0$ x 17]

OUTPUT

[4839587218]+[38845461065246]+[25832109]

[38850326484573]

[66]

[12]

[**3**]-[8-5-4-7-**3**]

It implies that primary healthcare center is among the right places to go for making health inquiries.

2-HEALTH-INTEGRATED CODE

Working From The First Dimension, We Have:

Input= $[O^1$ x Q] A Slide per Letter

INPUT = HEALTH

DATA

O -26

I - 6letters: 5, 4,3,2,1,0

Q-h= 7, e =4, a = 0, l = 11, t=19, h= 7

COMPUTING

$h[26^5 \times 7] + e[26^4 \times 4] + a[26^3 \times 0] + l[26^2 \times 11] + t[26^1 \times 19] + h[26^0 \times 7]$

OUTPUT IN FIGURES

[85005473]-this is the Cardinal value of the word 'health'

Hence, to derive *Health-Integrated Code*, the above cardinal values need to be reduced to a single-digit.

[85005473]+ [8+5+0+0+5+4+7+3]=32[3+2]=[**5**]

Interpretation Of Heath-Integrated Code

INPUT = DISEASES

COMPUTING

$d[26^7 \times 3] + i[26^6 \times 8] + s[26^5 \times 18] + e[26^4 \times 4] + a[26^3 \times 0] + s[26^2 \times 18] + e[26^1 \times 4] + s[26^0 \times 18]$

OUTPUT

[26782461698]

[59]

[14]

[5]-[5]-health-integrated code

It implies that diseases are among the major threats to human health.

INPUT = INFECTIONS

COMPUTING

$i[26^9 \times 8] + n[26^8 \times 13] + f[26^7 \times 5] + e[26^6 \times 4] + c[26^5 \times 2] + t[26^4 \times 19] + i[26^3 \times 8] + o[26^2 \times 14] + n[26^1 \times 13] + s[26^0 \times 18]$

OUTPUT

[46192208581004]

[50]

[5]-[5]-health-integrated code

It implies that infections are among the major threats to human health.

INPUT = TUMOR

COMPUTING

$t[26^4 \times 19] + u[26^3 \times 20] + m[26^2 \times 12] + o[26^1 \times 14] + r[26^0 \times 17]$

OUTPUT

[9042557]

[32]

[5]-[5]-health-integrated code

It implies that tumor is among the major threats to human health.

INPUT = DEATH

COMPUTING

$d[26^4 \times 3] + e[26^3 \times 4] + a[26^2 \times 0] + t[26^1 \times 19] + h[26^0 \times 7]$

OUTPUT

[1441733]

[23]

[5]-[5]-health-integrated code

It implies that death is among the major threats to human health.

INPUT = LIFE

COMPUTING

l[26^3 x 11] +i[26^2 x 8] + f[26^1 x 5] + e[26^0 x 4]

OUTPUT

[198878]

[41]

[5]-[5]-health-integrated code

It implies that life is among the major supports to human health.

INPUT = TREATMENT

COMPUTING

t[26^8 x 19] + r[26^7 x 17] + e[26^6 x 4] +a[26^5 x 0] + t[26^4 x 19] + m [26^3 x 12] +e[26^2 x 4] + n[26^1 x 13] + t[26^0 x 19]

OUTPUT

[4105499559557]

[68]

[14]

[5]-[5]-health-integrated code

It implies that treatment is among the major supports to human health.

INPUT = DOCTORS

COMPUTING

d[26^6 x 3] +o[26^5 x 14] + c[26^4 x 2] +t[26^3 x 19] +o[26^2 x 14] +

r[26^1 x 17] + s[26^0 x 18]

OUTPUT

[1094344412]

[41]

[5]-[5]-health-integrated code

It implies that doctors play a key role in taking care of the health of

human being

INPUT = PHARMACISTS

COMPUTING

p[26^{10} x 15]+h[26^9 x 7] + a[26^8 x 0] + r[26^7 x 17] + m[26^6 x 12]

+a[26^5 x 0] + c[26^4 x 2] +i[26^3 x 8] +s[26^2 x1 8] + t[26^1 x 19] +

s[26^0 x 18]

OUTPUT

[2155653209383016]

[59]

[14]

[5]-[5]-health-integrated code

It implies that pharmacists play a key role in taking care of the health

of human being.

INPUT = RADIOLOGIST

COMPUTING

r[26^{10} x 17]+a[26^9 x 0] + d[26^8 x 3] + i[26^7 x 8] + o[26^6 x 14]

+l$[26^5 \times 11]$ + o$[26^4 \times 14]$ +g$[26^3 \times 6]$ +i$[26^2 \times 8]$ + s$[26^1 \times 18]$ + t$[26^0 \times 19]$

OUTPUT

[2400535823807543]

[59]

[14]

[5]-[5]-health-integrated code

It implies that radiologists play a key role in taking care of the health of human being.

INPUT = SCIENTIST

COMPUTING

s$[26^8 \times 18]$ + c$[26^7 \times 2]$ + i$[26^6 \times 8]$ +e$[26^5 \times 4]$ + n$[26^4 \times 13]$ +t$[26^3 \times 19]$ +i$[26^2 \times 8]$ + s$[26^1 \times 18]$ + t$[26^0 \times 19]$

OUTPUT

[3777475914959]

[77]

[14]

[5]-[5]-health-integrated code

It implies that scientists play a key role in taking care of the health of human being.

INPUT = NURSE

COMPUTING

n$[26^4 \times 13]$ +u$[26^3 \times 20]$ +r$[26^2 \times 17]$ + s$[26^1 \times 18]$ + e$[26^0 \times 4]$

OUTPUT

[6304172]

[23]

[5]-[5]-health-integrated code

 It implies that nurses play a key role in taking care of the health of human being

CONCLUSION

Based on the health integrated code, 5 personnel form the network of health-care system:-doctors, pharmacists, radiologists, scientists and nurses

3-HEALTH-ORGAN OF INTEREST

The only organ whose well being is for the benefit of the whole body is the heart. When it falls sick all the other parts of the human body are at risk.

INPUT = HEART

COMPUTING

 $h[26^4 \times 7] + e[26^3 \times 4] + a[26^2 \times 0] + r[26^1 \times 17] + t[26^0 \times 19]$

OUTPUT

[3269597]-the cardinal value of heart

[41]

[5]-[5]-health-integrated code

It implies that the heart is the only organ that when become affected by a disease, all other structures inside the human body are at risk.

HEALTH-SAFETY PRECAUTIONS

There are 9 heath-safety precautions inscribed inside the heart of every individual, which if follow strictly, an individual will have nearly 100% chances of a healthy- life .There would be no medical burden on your health and your little source of income would be safe.

Heart –Segmented Code

From the above cardinal value of heart, we can deduce the heart segmented code to be:

[3269597]= **[3-2-6-9-5-7]-The Heart-Segmented Code**

VERIFICATION OF HEALTH-SAFETY PRECAUTIONS
[NO.1] **INPUT = ADEQUATE VENTILATION** **COMPUTING** $a[26^7 \times 0] + d[26^6 \times 3] + e[26^5 \times 4] + q[26^4 \times 16] + u[26^3 \times 20] + a[26^2 \times 0] + t[26^1 \times 19] + e[26^0 \times 4] \ / + / v[26^{10} \times 21] + e[26^9 \times 4] + n[26^8 \times 13] + t[26^7 \times 19] + i[26^6 \times 8] + l[26^5 \times 11] + a[26^4 \times 0] + t[26^3 \times 19] + i[26^2 \times 8] + o[26^1 \times 14] + n[26^0 \times 13]$

OUTPUT

[981936466]+[2989096982030705]

[2989097963967171]

[93]

[12]

[**3**]- [**3**-2-6-9-5-7]

Hence, adequate ventilation is among the fundamentals of healthy -life

[NO.2]

INPUT = HAND CLEANING

COMPUTING

h[26^3 x 7] +a[26^2 x 0] + n[26^1 x 13] + d[26^0 x 3] /+/
c[26^7 x 2] + l[26^6 x 11] +e[26^5 x 4] + a[26^4 x 0] +n[26^3 x 13] +i[26^2 x 8] + n[26^1 x 13] + g[26^0 x 6]

OUTPUT

[123373]+[19509453632]

[19509577005]

[48]

[12]

[**3**]- [**3**-2-6-9-5-7]

Hence, hand cleaning is among the fundamentals of healthy –life

[NO.3]

INPUT = DIET

COMPUTING

$d[26^3 \times 7] + i[26^2 \times 0] + e[26^1 \times 13] + t[26^0 \times 3]$

OUTPUT

[58259]

[29]

[11]

[**2**]- [3-**2**-6-9-5-7]

Hence, diet is among the fundamentals of healthy -life

[NO.4]

INPUT = EXERCISE

COMPUTING

$e[26^7 \times 4] + x[26^6 \times 23] + e[26^5 \times 4] + r[26^4 \times 17] + c[26^3 \times 2] + i[26^2 \times 8] + s[26^1 \times 18] + e[26^0 \times 4]$

OUTPUT

[39287638680]

[60]

[**6**]- [3-2-**6**-9-5-7]

Hence, exercise is among the fundamentals of healthy – life

[NO.5]

INPUT =SLEEPING

COMPUTING

s[26^7 x18]+ l[26^6 x 11] +e[26^5 x 4] + e[26^4 x 4] + p[26^3 x 15] +i[26^2 x 8] + n[26^1 x 13] + g[26^0 x 6]

OUTPUT

[148020279504]

[42]

[**6**]- [3-2-**6**-9-5-7]

Hence, sleeping is among the fundamentals of healthy - life

[NO.6]

INPUT = MOUTH CARE

COMPUTING

m[26^4 x 12] + o[26^3 x 14] +u[26^2 x 20] + t[26^1 x 19] + h[26^0 x 7] /+/c[26^3 x 2] +a[26^2 x 0] + r[26^1 x 17] + e[26^0 x 4]

OUTPUT

[5743797]+[35598]

[5779395]

[45]

[9]

[**9**]- [3-2-6-**9**-5-7]

Hence, mouth care is among the fundamentals of healthy -life

[NO.7]

INPUT = PROPER ENVIRONMENTAL SANITATION

COMPUTING

p[26^5 x 15] + r[26^4 x 17] + o[26^3 x 14] +p[26^2 x 15] + e[26^1 x 4] + r[26^0 x 17] /+/e[26^{12} x 4]+n[26^{11} x 13]+v[26^{10} x21]+ i[26^9 x 8] + r[26^8 x 17] + o[26^7 x 14] + n[26^6 x 13] +m[26^5 x 12] + e[26^4 x 4] +n[26^3 x 13] +t[26^2 x 19] + a[26^1 x 0] + l[26^0 x 11]/+/ s[26^9 x 18] + a[26^8 x 0] + n[26^7 x 13] + i[26^6 x 8] +t[26^5 x 19] + a[26^4 x 0] +t[26^3 x 19] +i[26^2 x 8] + o[26^1 x 14] + n[26^0 x 13]

OUTPUT

[186245557]+[432441916681713599]+

[97838177165937]

[432539755045125093]

[72]

[**9**]- [3-2-6-**9**-5-7]

Hence, proper environmental sanitation is among the fundamentals of healthy –life

[NO.8]

INPUT = GOOD CLOTHING

COMPUTING

g[26^3 x 6] +o[26^2 x 14] + o[26^1 x 14] + d[26^0 x 3] /+/

c[26^7 x 2] + l[26^6 x 11] +o[26^5 x 14] + t[26^4 x 19]

+h[26^3 x 7] +i[26^2 x 8] + n[26^1 x 13] + g[26^0 x 6]

OUTPUT

[115287]+[19636844480]

[19636959767]

[68]

[14]

[**5**]- [3-2-6-9-**5**-7]

Hence, good clothing is among the fundamentals of healthy -life

[NO.9]

INPUT = CARE OF PERINEAL AREA

COMPUTING

c[26^3 x 2] +a[26^2 x 0] + r[26^1 x 17] + e[26^0 x 4] /+/

o[26^1 x 14] + f[26^0 x 5] /+/ p[26^7 x 15] + e[26^6 x 4]

+r[26^5 x 17] + i[26^4 x 8] +n[26^3 x 13] +e[26^2 x 4] +

a[26^1 x 0] + l[26^0 x 11] /+/ a[26^3 x 0] +r[26^2 x 17] +

$e[26^1 \times 4] + a[26^0 \times 0]$

OUTPUT

[35598]+[369]+[121918686147   ]+[11596]

[121918733710]

[43]

[7]

[5]- [3-2-6-9-5-<u>7</u>]

Hence, care of perineal area is among the fundamentals of healthy -life

The 9 Health-Safety Precautions Are:

1-Adequate Ventilation

2-Hand Cleaning

3-Diet

4-Exercise

5-Sleeping

6-Mouth Care

7-Proper Environmental Sanitation

8-Good Clothing

ADEQUATE VENTILATION

SIX WAYS POOR VENTILATION CAN AFFECT YOUR EMPLOYEES' HEALTHADAPTED FROM AN ARTICLE WRITTEN IN FSP BUSINESS, 12 JUNE 2013

Poor ventilation is a hazard. And like all hazards, it poses a risk to your employees' health and you must eliminate or control it at all costs. If you don't, it'll slow down productivity in your workplace and result in increased sick leave. But these aren't the only consequences. Read on to discover the six ways poor ventilation will affect your employees. Then find out the easy solution, that you can use to protect your employee's health.

Proper office ventilation is needed to remove unpleasant smells and excessive moisture, introduce outside air to keep interior building air circulated, and to prevent stagnation of the indoor air.

That's why you must ventilate your workplace either by natural (eg. solar) or mechanical (eg. aircon, fans) means.   Failure to do so will increase health and safety risks to your employees.

Not only does poor ventilation affect the physical health of your employees, but psychological effects like stress also rise when your employees are constantly exposed to the effects of poor ventilation. The consequences of this can be dire.

Poor ventilation affects your employees in these six ways:

Here's a look at some of the consequences of poor ventilation to your employees:

High levels of carbon dioxide and low levels of oxygen can cause fatigue and affect your employee's ability to concentrate.

Build up of chemical and biological contaminants that cause poor indoor air quality.   Poor indoor air quality can lead to employees suffering from headaches, fatigue, hypersensitivity and allergies, sinus congestion dizziness, shortness of breath, coughing and nausea.

Extreme temperature in the office causes fatigue,

discomfort and distraction and can increase accidents in the workplace as a result.

Low humidity can cause a dry throat, dry skin and static electricity build-up. High humidity contributes to bacterial and mould growth. This can make your employees very sick.

Excessive and irritating workplace odours cause discomfort and affect concentration. For example, ammonia and chlorine.

Poor ventilation causes Sick Building Syndrome (SBS). The symptoms include irritation of eyes, nose and throat, headaches, fatigue, and a susceptibility to colds and flu. Symptoms tend to be less severe away from the workplace.

There you have it.Knowing how poor ventilation can affect your employees' health will ensure that you make ventilation a top priority on your company's health and safety list. Find out how the Solazone solar ventilators can improve the air quality in your building, at surprisingly little cost.

RELATED SOURCE

http://www.solazone.com.au/air-heating-ventilation/

HAND CLEANING

SHOW ME THE SCIENCE - WHY WASH YOUR HANDS?

ESPAÑOL (SPANISH)

Keeping hands clean is one of the most important steps we can take to avoid getting sick and spreading germs to others. Many diseases and conditions are spread by not washing hands with soap and clean, running water.

How germs get onto hands and make people sick Feces (poop) from people or animals is an important source of germs like Salmonella, E. coli O157, and norovirus that cause diarrhea, and it can spread some respiratory infections like adenovirus and hand-foot-mouth disease. These kinds of germs can get onto hands after people use the toilet or change a diaper, but also in less obvious ways, like after handling raw meats that have invisible amounts of animal poop on them. A single gram of human feces—which is about the weight of a paper clip—can contain one trillion germs 1. Germs can also get onto hands if people touch any object that has germs on it because someone coughed or sneezed on it or was touched by some other contaminated object. When these germs get onto hands and are not washed off, they can be passed from person to person and make people sick. Washing hands prevents illnesses and spread of infections to others

Handwashing with soap removes germs from hands. This helps prevent infections because:

People frequently touch their eyes, nose, and mouth without even realizing it. Germs can get into the body through the eyes, nose and mouth and make us sick.

Germs from unwashed hands can get into foods and drinks while people prepare or consume them. Germs can multiply in some types of foods or drinks, under certain conditions, and make people sick.

Germs from unwashed hands can be transferred to other objects, like handrails, table tops, or toys, and then transferred to another person's hands.

Removing germs through handwashing therefore helps prevent diarrhea and respiratory infections and may even help prevent skin and eye infections.

Teaching people about handwashing helps them and their communities stay healthy. Handwashing education in the community:

Reduces the number of people who get sick with diarrhea by 23-40% 2, 3, 6

Reduces diarrheal illness in people with weakened immune systems by 58% 4

Reduces respiratory illnesses, like colds, in the general population by 16-21% 3, 5

Reduces absenteeism due to gastrointestinal illness in schoolchildren by 29-57% 7

Not washing hands harms children around the world

About 1.8 million children under the age of 5 die each year from diarrheal diseases and pneumonia, the top two killers of young children around the world

Handwashing with soap could protect about 1 out of every 3 young children who get sick with diarrhea 2, 3 and almost 1 out of 5 young children with respiratory infections like pneumonia 3, 5.

Although people around the world clean their hands with water, very few use soap to wash their hands. Washing hands with soap removes germs much more effectively 9.

Handwashing education and access to soap in schools

can help improve attendance 10, 11, 12.

Good handwashing early in life may help improve child development in some settings 13.

Estimated global rates of handwashing after using the toilet are only 19% 6.

Handwashing helps battle the rise in antibiotic resistance

Preventing sickness reduces the amount of antibiotics people use and the likelihood that antibiotic resistance will develop. Handwashing can prevent about 30% of diarrhea-related sicknesses and about 20% of respiratory infections (e.g., colds) 2, 5. Antibiotics often are prescribed unnecessarily for these health issues 14. Reducing the number of these infections by washing hands frequently helps prevent the overuse of antibiotics—the single most important factor leading to antibiotic resistance around the world. Handwashing can also prevent people from getting sick with germs that are already resistant to antibiotics and that can be difficult to treat.

RELATED SOURCE

https://www.cdc.gov/handwashing/why-handwashing.html

Eat your food like medicine,

Else you have to eat your medicine as food

You may find this statement inimical but, it is true.

When we hear 'diet and health problems' is not always

'obesity'. There are various different health problems

related to diet have discovered in skinny people too.

Diet or the nutrition is one of the fundamental necessity

of a human body to stay healthy and work with the

enthusiasm all day long.

It will not merely help you stay but prevent many

chronic diseases such as diabetes, heart diseases,

obesity, eating disorders, and osteoporosis. Here are

some diet tactics to keep you going.

Need For Good Food

Not food but the good food is one of the basic needs of

healthy human beings. Now, how to define the good

food? The food which is full of the nutrients essential

such as protein, vitamins, minerals, carbohydrates,

fibers, etc. You must make sure your everyday food

contains at least the required amount of the healthy

ingredients.

Eating Too Much Or Too Less

It is one of the questions asked in scores because too little food may lead to malnutrition and too much to obesity. Other eating disorders are anorexia nervosa, bulimia, binge-eating disorder. Then what is the best quantity we should consume?

Many a time our diet get affected due to the emotional, social, physical, mental, and environmental conditions. This is perilous to your overall health hence as mentioned earlier we need to take our food like medicine. In proper quantity, on scheduled time, and without fail.

Poor Nutrition? How Does It Affect Us?

Poor nutrition is one of the grave concerns in many corners of the world, particularly in India.

On the Global Hunger Index India is on place 67 among the 80 nations having the worst hunger situation which is worse than nations such as North Korea or Sudan. 25% of all hungry people worldwide live in India. Since 1990 there have been some improvements for children but the proportion of hungry in the population has increased. In India 44% of children under the age of 5 are underweight. 72% of infants and 52% of married women have anemia. Research has conclusively shown that malnutrition during pregnancy causes the child to have increased risk of future diseases, physical retardation, and reduced cognitive abilities.

Therefore, it is essential to take care of our nutrition as well as the people around by any possible means to help the nation's health mission.

Overeating And Problems

Obesity is an obvious flip side of malnutrition. Where the number of children dying underweight, obesity emerged as the chief health issue.

According to WHO, worldwide, at least 2.8 million people die each year as a result of being overweight or obese, and an estimated 35.8 million (2.3%) of global DALYs are caused by overweight or obesity.

Obesity has reached epidemic proportions in India in the 21st century, with morbid obesity affecting 5% of the country's population.

These demises arose due to the diseases fall down the road with obesity. Such as hypertension, type 2 diabetes, cholesterol, osteoporosis, cancer, and other heart diseases.

Modern Diet (Junk Food) And Its Impact

In the 21st century, youth is under this giant problem they couldn't disregard and resulted in the increased number of demises. Junk food, for instance, pizza, burgers, cookies, fried pies, etc impact your overall health. It not merely affect your heart or stomach but deteriorate your health from head to toe.

Junk food contains calories, fats and sodium like health hazardous contents in inept quantity.

Frequently occurring headache, depression, acne or hindrance in breath could have resulted from your cravings for junk food. This is not it, chronic diseases such as heart disease or stroke, high cholesterol, weight gain (probably your chief concern these days), high blood pressure can also have arisen from junk food.

Not mere one or two but scores of problems or simply every health issue is due to ignorance of diet.

There are many such undesired health problems you may need to face if you ignore your diet. Hence, one and all should include fruits, vegetables, grains and nuts in the diet.

Eat What Your Body Needs, Not What Your

Temptation!!

RELATED SOURCE

https://www.medclique.org/nutrition-and-diet/poor-diet-health-problems/

EXERCISE

Physical Inactivity

Muscle Atrophy And Joint Pain

The process of your muscles breaking down or wasting away is the medical definition of muscle atrophy.According to the American Council on Exercise, muscles begin to break down when they aren't exercised to their full capacity. You gain fattier tissue after your muscle has been broken down as well as lose lean muscle. As a result of the loss of muscle or muscle atrophy, your metabolism can slow and you can begin to gain even more fat.

Arthritic joints can stiffen and theadjoining tissue can weaken after long periods of inactivity

There is an increased risk for low back pain for those who do not exercise regularly, especially during times when a person may suddenly have to perform stressful, unfamiliar activities.

Weight Regain After Dieting

Lack of exercise may lead you to regain weight that you have lost, as most are tempted to stop exercising once they have reached goal weight. Exercise is the most highly recommended way to prevent weight regain, according to the National Heart, Lung, and Blood Institute.

Depression

Inactivity, research suggests, may have a detrimental effect on your mental health.[4] There has been shown to be an association between lack of exercise and depression and a lower sense of general well-being, according to research from the American College of Sports

Cardiac Decline

According to the American Council on Exercise, because your heart is also a muscle, your heart begins to rapidly decline in cardiovascular fitness when you don't get enough exercise. Fat will begin to attack the heart, even though it won't waste away like your arm or leg muscles. Heart disease, hardening of the arteries, and atherosclerosis are all conditions that can develop from this. Fat deposits can enter the valves and chambers of a person's heart, which can be fatal, as fatty deposits will begin to build up in your arteries from lack of exercise.

Because exercise helps to keep blood pressure and cholesterol at healthy levels , about 35 percent of heart disease deaths are due to lack of exercise, according to The New York State Department.

Increased Visceral Fat

Fat that becomes entrapped deep inside your abdomen is known as visceral fat.6   This visceral fat can secrete dangerous hormones and cause health problems such as gallbladder difficulties, heart disease, and metabolic syndrome, making it very toxic. You may also be at risk of developing breast cancer or insulin resistance, which can lead to diabetes due to the toxic hormones produced by these fat cells. If you have visceral fat you also put yourself at an increased risk of developing colorectal cancer.

Intestinal Effects

According to KidsHealth.org, constipation can be caused by lack of exercise. Your body's digestion process slows when you don't exercise, causing constipation. Exercise itself helps your body pass solid waste and promotes digestion.

Diabetes

Deaths related to diabetes and diabetes itself are strongly associated with lack of exercise, according to research published in the July 2005 issue of "Diabetes Care".

RELATED SOURCE

https://www.livewellwinona.org/facts/risk-factors-related-illnesses/physical-inactivity/

SLEEPING

What Happens to Your Body When You Don't Get Enough Sleep?

If you eat well and exercise regularly but don't get at least seven hours of sleep every night, you may undermine all your other efforts.

Sleep disorders expert Harneet Walia, MD, says it's important to focus on getting enough sleep, something many of us lack. "First and foremost, we need to make sleep a priority," she says. "We always recommend a good diet and exercise to everyone. Along the same lines, we need to focus on sleep as well."

How Much Sleep Do You Actually Need?

Everyone feels better after a good night's rest. But now, thanks to a report from the National Sleep Foundation, you can aim for a targeted sleep number tailored to your age.

The foundation based its report on two years of research. Published in a recent issue of the foundation's journal Sleep Health, the report updates previous sleep recommendations. It breaks them into nine age-specific categories with a range for each, which allows for individual differences:

Older adults, 65+ years: 7-8 hours

Adults, 26-64 years: 7-9 hours

Young adults, 18-25 years: 7-9 hours

Teenagers, 14-17 years: 8-10 hours

School-age children, 6-13 years: 9-11 hours

Preschool children, 3-5 years: 10-13 hours

Toddlers, 1-2 years: 11-14 hours

Infants, 4-11 months: 12-15 hours

Newborns, 0-3 months: 14-17 hours

Dr. Walia says there's evidence that genetic, behavioral and environmental factors help determine how much sleep an individual needs for the best health and daily performance.

But a minimum of seven hours of sleep is a step in the right direction to improve your health, she says.

<u>What Happens When You Don't Get Enough Sleep?</u>

Your doctor urges you to get enough sleep for good reason, Dr. Walia says. Shorting yourself on shut-eye has a negative impact on your health in many ways:

Short-term problems can include:

Lack of alertness: Even missing as little as 1.5 hours can have an impact, research shows.

Impaired memory: Lack of sleep can affect your ability to think and to remember and process information.

Relationship stress: It can make you feel moody, and you can become more likely to have conflicts with others.

Quality of life: You may become less likely to participate in normal daily activities or to exercise.

Greater likelihood for car accidents: Drowsy driving accounts for thousands of crashes, injuries and fatalities each year, according to the National Highway Traffic Safety Administration.

If you continue to operate without enough sleep, you may see more long-term and serious health problems. Some of the most serious potential problems associated with chronic sleep deprivation are high blood pressure, diabetes, heart attack, heart failure or stroke. Other potential problems include obesity, depression and lower sex drive.

Chronic sleep deprivation can even affect your appearance. Over time, it can lead to premature wrinkling and dark circles under the eyes. Also, research links a lack of sleep to an increase of the stress hormone cortisol in the body. Cortisol can break down collagen, the protein that keeps skin smooth.

Make Time For Downtime

"In our society, nowadays, people aren't getting enough sleep. They put sleep so far down on their priority list because there are so many other things to do – family, personal and work life," Dr. Walia says. "These are challenges, but if people understand how important adequate sleep is, it makes a huge difference."

RELATED SOURCE

https://health.clevelandclinic.org/happens-body-dont-get-enough-sleep/

MOUTH CARE

Although you probably understand that poor dental care can lead to cavities, did you know that other, more serious health problems can also result from poor oral care? The truth is that if you don't take proper care of your teeth, you could face far more serious consequences than a simple toothache or some unsightly stains.

The Mayo Clinic, as well as a report from ABC News, highlight some major areas of concern:

Cardiovascular disease: In a nutshell, this means heart disease. The bacteria from inflammation of the gums and periodontal disease can enter your bloodstream and travel to the arteries in the heart and cause atherosclerosis (hardening of the arteries). Atherosclerosis causes plaque to develop on the inner walls of arteries which thicken and this decreases or may block blood flow through the body. This can cause an increased risk of heart attack or stroke. The inner lining of the heart can also become infected and inflamed a condition known as endocarditis.

Dementia: The bacteria from gingivitis may enter the brain through either nerve channels in the head or through the bloodstream, that might even lead to the development of Alzheimer's disease.

Respiratory infections: The Journal of Periodontology warns that gum disease could cause you to get infections in your lungs, including pneumonia. While the connection might not be completely obvious at first, think of what might happen from breathing in bacteria from infected teeth and gums over a long period of time.

Diabetic complications: Inflammation of the gum tissue and periodontal disease can make it harder to control your blood sugar and make your diabetes symptoms worse. Diabetes sufferers are also more susceptible to periodontal disease, making proper dental care even more important for those with this disease.

As you can see, brushing and flossing keep more than your pearly whites healthy -- they might also prevent serious illnesses. Poor dental care is also a possible factor in other conditions, such as immune system disorders, weak bones, and problems with pregnancy and low birth weight.

Establish Good Hygiene Habits

The message is clear: Practicing proper dental care is important in many ways you might not have thought of before. Encourage your family to practice good oral hygiene by brushing after every meal with a fluoride toothpaste, flossing daily and using a mouth rinse to kill bacteria. You should also visit a dental professional regularly for cleanings and the prevention and treatment of cavities. Doing so can protect more than just your teeth -- it can save your life!

NOTE:

This article is intended to promote understanding of and knowledge about general oral health topics. It is not intended to be a substitute for professional advice, diagnosis or treatment. Always seek the advice of your dentist or other qualified healthcare provider with any questions you may have regarding a medical condition or treatment.

RELATED SOURCE

PROPER ENVIRONMENTAL SANITATION

Poor Sanitation Threatens Public Health

6 in 10 Africans remain without access to proper toilet

WHO/UNICEF

20 MARCH 2008 | GENEVA

- Sixty-two per cent of Africans do not have access to an improved sanitation facility -- a proper toilet -- which separates human waste from human contact, according to the WHO/UNICEF Joint Monitoring Programme for Water Supply and Sanitation. A global report will be published later this year, however, preliminary data on the situation in Africa was released today as part of World Water Day 2008. The Day, built around the theme that "Sanitation matters," seeks to draw attention to the plight of some 2.6 billion people around the world who live without access to a toilet at home and thus are vulnerable to a range of health risks.

"Sanitation is a cornerstone of public health," said WHO Director-General Dr Margaret Chan. "Improved sanitation contributes enormously to human health and well-being, especially for girls and women. We know that simple, achievable interventions can reduce the risk of contracting diarrhoeal disease by a third."

Although WHO and UNICEF estimate that 1.2 billion people worldwide gained access to improved sanitation between 1990 and 2004, an estimated 2.6 billion people - including 980 million children – had no toilets at home. If current trends continue, there will still be 2.4 billion people without basic sanitation in 2015, and the children among them will continue to pay the price in lost lives, missed schooling, in disease, malnutrition and poverty.

"Nearly 40% of the world's population lacks access to toilets, and the dignity and safety that they provide," said Ann M. Veneman, UNICEF Executive Director. "The absence of adequate sanitation has a serious impact on health and social development, especially for children. Investments in improving sanitation will accelerate progress towards the Millennium Development Goals and save lives."

Using proper toilets and hand washing - preferably with soap - prevents the transfer of bacteria, viruses and parasites found in human excreta which otherwise contaminate water resources, soil and food. This contamination is a major cause of diarrhoea, the second biggest killer of children in developing countries, and leads to other major diseases such as cholera, schistosomiasis, and trachoma.

Improving access to sanitation is a critical step towards reducing the impact of these diseases. It also helps create physical environments that enhance safety, dignity and self-esteem. Safety issues are particularly important for women and children, who otherwise risk sexual harassment and assault when defecating at night and in secluded areas.

Also, improving sanitation facilities and promoting hygiene in schools benefits both learning and the health of children. Child-friendly schools that offer private and separate toilets for boys and girls, as well as facilities for hand washing with soap, are better equipped to attract and retain students, especially girls. Where such facilities are not available, girls are often withdrawn from school when they reach puberty.

In health-care facilities, safe disposal of human waste of patients, staff and visitors is an essential environmental health measure. This intervention can contribute to the reduction of the transmission of health-care associated infections which affect 5% to 30% of patients.

"The focus on sanitation is fundamental to human beings," says Pasquale Steduto, UN-Water chairman. "The MDG target on sanitation is seriously lagging behind schedule. The entire UN System has a shared responsibility in mobilizing concrete actions towards its achievement; investments must increase immediately."

UN-Water is the coordinating mechanism of the UN agencies, programmes and funds that play a significant role in tackling global water and sanitation concerns.

World Water Day provides an opportunity to draw attention to the International Year of Sanitation 2008, a year in which the UN General Assembly in December 2006 has called for a focus on addressing sanitation and hygiene problems.

The International Year of Sanitation 2008 aims to raise the profile of sanitation issues on the international agenda and to accelerate progress towards meeting the

Millennium Development Goal target of reducing by half the proportion of people living without access to improved sanitation by 2015. Within the UN system, the focal point for the International Year of Sanitation is the United Nations Department of Economic and Social Affairs, in collaboration with the UN-Water Task Force on Sanitation.

Sanitation is not a dirty word. Sanitation matters.

RELATED SOURCE

https://www.who.int/mediacentre/news/releases/2008/pr08/en/

GOOD COTHING

How tight clothing can be harmful?

[1]Many people like to wear clothes which are trendy. Fashions and designs of clothes keep on changing. Maybe, this is because people want to wear something different and smart. The entire industry involved in designing, manufacturing and marketing clothes keeps this trend alive.

Somehow tight clothes have also entered the pattern of what is fashionable and many people can be seen wearing tight skinny jeans and body hugging dresses. Tight clothes in any form; whether jeans or tops or undergarments s are harmful.

Very tight jeans can compress the nerves of the thighs causing pain, tingling and numbness in the thighs and or legs. Cramps in the calf muscles can occur due to wearing very tight pantaloons or jeans. Muscle pain can occur due to constriction of the blood vessels hampering blood supply and also due to the pressure on the muscles and soft tissues.

The problem of heart burn i.e. burning sensation in the chest increases by wearing tight clothes. This happens because the pressure on the abdomen forces the flow of acid upwards causing heart burn.

Low blood pressure can result from wearing tight jeans, because the blood circulation and return of blood to the heart is impaired. One feels dizzy on standing due to low blood pressure and this can lead to fainting.

In women very tight clothes are known to cause sterility. This is more so in those who have been using tight clothes since teen years.

Tight clothes have been implicated in causing endometriosis a condition causing chronic abdominal pain in women. Recent researchers have postulated that chronic abdominal pain in women of higher class during the Victorian era could have been because of wearing clothes which were very tight across the waist.

Tight brassieres are a known cause for breast cancer in women. Tight clothes also increase the warmth and dampness in any part of the body making the part more susceptible to fungal infections. Fungal infections over genital parts and around in women have been known to result from tight undergarments. Pregnant women are advised to wear lose comfortable clothes because of multiple health hazards. Tightness around the abdomen is harmful for pregnant women as well.

In men wearing tight undergarments and or pantaloons can increase the warmth in the scrotal region and reduce sperm production. In extreme cases, it can result in infertility. Men can also suffer from fungal infections on and around genital parts due to tight undergarments, though it is more common in women.

Thus it can be seen clearly that there are multiple harmful effects of wearing tight clothes but absolutely no advantage. Therefore before an individual decides to wear and buy a tight fitting trendy looking dress, he or she should be aware of the harm it can cause

RELATED SOURCE

https://www.newtimes.co.rw/section/read/89410

[2] The pressures of continually evolving fashion have led both men and women into wearing ill fitting clothing. Here are some documented health problems from wearing clothes that are too tight:

- Tingling Thigh Syndrome: Although rarely permanent, individuals who wear their jeans too tight can experience nerve problems called meralgia paresthetic. If your thigh tingles with no explanation, then it's probably time to stop wearing extra tight clothes for your own good.

- Yeast Infection: When women's pubic areas are kept tightly under wraps by clothing such as tight jeans or underwear especially g-strings, the area becomes very warm and moist. This makes it a breeding ground for bacteria and, as a result, can cause yeast infections and also urinary tract infections.

.-Back Pain: When trousers are low riding and too tight nerve compression in the back could occur and this leads to severe low back pain.

- Fainting: Although the girdle isn't as popular as it used to be, body magic and the like have taken its place. Tight clothing can restrict our ability to fully expand our lungs making breathing shallow and decreasing oxygen intake and this can lead to fainting.

- Heartburn: Tight pressure against your stomach can increase abdominal pressure, causing acid to go back into your esophagus, resulting in heart burn and acid reflux.

- Abdominal Pain/Constipation: Tight trousers can slow down the digestive process.

- Headaches/Blurred Vision: Wearing button down shirts that are too tight in the collar or ties that are tied too tightly can decrease proper circulation to the brain and head.

- Infertility: Tight fitting trousers can lead to bladder

problems, twisted testicles, low sperm count and even infertility.

So, next time you are tempted to buy an extremely tight garment, think twice. You might be putting your health at risk!

RELATED SOURCE

http://www.informationng.com/2013/04/tight-clothes-can-have-a-damaging-effect-on-your-health-doctors-say.html

[3] <u>Negative Effects of Tight Clothes on Pregnant Women</u>

Heartburn

The California Pacific Medical Center's Women & Infants Center points out that wearing tight-fitting clothes, especially at the waist, can lead to heartburn. Heartburn or acid reflux are common discomforts during pregnancy. These occur due to digestive slowness from an increase in progesterone in the body during pregnancy. When the stomach contents sit longer in the stomach due to this slowness, the risk of the contents flowing upwards increases. The fullness in the abdomen from the growing uterus, amniotic sac and baby can put pressure on the stomach and force the contents back up the chest too. The pressure from tight clothing can push on the stomach and force the contents upwards, creating heartburn.

Yeast Infection

The American Pregnancy Association suggests another effect of wearing tight, unbreathable clothing is increased vaginal yeast infections. Pregnant women experience an increase in vaginal secretions during pregnancy. This, combined with tight underwear, can create the perfect environment to allow yeast that naturally occurs in the vagina to overproduce and cause an infection.

Pain

Wearing tight-fitting clothes can cause pain in a number of areas of the body during pregnancy. This includes the abdomen, chest and arms. A woman's bra size can increase both in the elastic around the middle and the cup itself. Tight-fitting bras can cause pain in the breasts, under the arms and the back. As the woman nears labor, the breasts may be even more susceptible to pain or complications from tight-fitting bras. This is due to the breasts preparing to lactate when the baby is born. Putting pressure in one area of the breast too long can cause the milk ducts to become clogged even before a woman is breastfeeding. The result can be pain, redness and a knot.

Reduced Circulation

Wearing tight-fitting clothes, whether pregnant or not, can slow circulation in the body. In early pregnancy the woman's blood vessels expand in preparation for the increased blood volume that develops to provide for the placenta and baby. Before the blood volume increases to fill the vessels, a woman can experience hypotension, or low blood pressure, easily. Examples of this include standing up quickly from a kneeling, sitting or lying position. Tight clothes in the limbs, such as the arms and thighs, can cut off blood circulation and create a numbness or tingling sensation.

RELATED SOURCE

https://www.google.com/search?q=effect+of+tight+cl othes+during+pregnancy

[4] Tight Clothes During Pregnancy

Bras

One of the first things you might notice when you get

pregnant is a swelling and aching in your breasts. They are getting ready to feed your baby. As they grow, you may find the pain increasing under the tight environment of your old bras. It's time to invest in a new bra or two. If you are early in your pregnancy and worried about how much more they might grow, you can invest in one or two simple or convertible styles that you wear every day with every outfit. Look for a nursing bra with padding in a size bigger than what you currently need. When that bra starts getting tight as you grow, you can remove the padding for a little more space. That bra with padding will work again later if your breasts shrink a bit.

Pants

Pants and shorts are pesky clothing options during pregnancy. Your belly will pop out within the first few months, expanding your waist line. It won't be long before your jeans, dress pants and other snapping or zipping items won't close. Pressing yourself into tight clothes during pregnancy can aggravate your heart burn or exacerbate your varicose veins. Before you give up and throw on your husband's sweatpants, shop for pants at your local maternity store. You will find some low-rise options that will tuck nicely under your belly. These will still be wearable for weeks or months after you give birth. The bands are designed to fit around your belly; long blouses help cover your belly.

Dresses

If you are lucky, or unlucky, enough to be pregnant during the heat of summer, dresses will be your best friend. You can choose casual or formal options, so you can prance around in dresses every day. If wrap styles and sheath options are too tight around your stomach, looking for flowing and baby-doll options. These may be tighter around your breasts, for a sexy feminine look, and spill over your belly. You can show off that baby bump without wrapping it like a mummy.

RELATED SOURCE

https://www.modernmom.com/2d6cc2d2-051f-11e2-9d62-404062497d7e.html

CARE OF PERINEAL AREA

Healthy Hygiene to Prevent Yeast Infections

Vaginal yeast infections are common. In fact, most

women will have a vaginal yeast infection at some point in their lives.

"**Yeast Infection** is the second most common vaginal infection in women," says Lisa M. Krikorian, nurse practitioner in the gynecology clinic at The Lahey Hospital & Medical Center in Burlington, Mass. Bacterial vaginosis is the most common.

The organism that causes yeast infections is a fungus, Candida albicans, that normally lives in and around your vagina as well as in your digestive tract and on your skin. Much of the time, candida coexists peacefully with the other organisms that live in and on your body. These microorganisms are known as your normal flora. When something upsets the balance of your normal flora, one organism can get out of control, multiply too much, and cause an infection.

"Yeast grows best in a moist, dark, warm environment," says Krikorian. "Once you understand that, yeast infection causes make sense."

What Causes Yeast to Grow?

Some yeast infection causes can be harder to control than others. These include conditions that can upset the balance of your normal flora, like taking antibiotics or birth control pills, being pregnant, or having an illness.

Other yeast infection causes are due to excess irritation or moisture in the vaginal area. "These types of yeast infection causes can be controlled by practicing good feminine hygiene and taking some simple steps to avoid creating an environment that yeast likes to grow in," Krikorian says.

How Feminine Hygiene Helps Prevent Yeast Infection

Preventing yeast infections begins with taking good care of yourself — getting enough rest, avoiding stress, and eating a healthy diet. If you have diabetes, keep your blood sugar under control. Uncontrolled blood sugar levels can increase your likelihood of yeast infections and may make it harder to get rid of them. If you take antibiotics or birth control pills, ask your doctor if you should take probiotics to protect your "good" bacteria so that yeast won't overwhelm the vaginal area. In addition, good feminine hygiene helps prevent an environment that's suitable for yeast growth.

Practice these feminine hygiene tips to help prevent yeast infections:

1. Stay clean and dry.

Avoid cleaning your genital area with soap. Instead, rinse thoroughly with water only and dry completely with a soft towel. If wanted, you may use a mild soap. Change out of a wet bathing suit right after swimming. Change out of workout clothes and take a shower immediately after exercising.

Always wipe front to back.

2. Reduce natural moisture.

Wear loose-fitting underwear and pants. Leave some room for air flow.

Wear absorbent cotton or silk underwear instead of nylon or other synthetic fabrics.

3. Avoid using feminine hygiene products that can disrupt the natural bacteria balance.

Avoid douching.

Don't use feminine hygiene sprays, powders, and fragrances.

4. Bathe smartly.

Stay out of hot tubs.

Limit your time soaking in a hot bath.

Thoroughly rinse after using products like bath salts.

5. Take extra care during menstruation.

Keep your genital area clean.

Use pads instead of tampons if you are prone to yeast infections.

If you use tampons, change them frequently.

Avoid scented pads or tampons.

6. Practice safe sex.

Always use condoms if you aren't in a committed relationship.

"If you have a yeast infection, you should avoid intercourse until your symptoms clear. Vaginal sex can make symptoms of itching, soreness, and dryness worse," says Krikorian.

In general, practicing healthy habits — getting enough rest, eating a healthy diet, and taking care of your feminine hygiene — helps reduce your risk of a yeast infection. If you experience frequent vaginal infections, talk to your doctor about other possible causes.

RELATED SOURCE

https://www.everydayhealth.com/hs/yeast-infection/healthy-hygiene-to-prevent-yeast-infection/

[2]Personal Hygiene For Women

The vagina is able to clean itself no special care is

needed, other than washing the external genitals. Do not put anything like douches into the vagina, as the delicate skin can be damaged. Here are some personal hygiene suggestions for women:

Menstruation - wash your body, including your genital area, in the same way as you always do. Change tampons and sanitary napkins regularly, at least four to five times a day. Always wash your hands before and after handling a tampon or pad.

Cystitis - is an infection of the bladder. This is a common condition for sexually active young women. Urinating after sexual intercourse can help to flush out any bacteria that may be in the urethra and bladder.

Thrush - some soaps and detergents can irritate the skin of the vagina, and make thrush infections more likely. Some people find that they often get thrush when they use antibiotics. Use mild soap and unperfumed toilet paper. Avoid tight, synthetic underwear. Try cotton underwear, and change regularly. There is medical treatment for thrush, so talk to your doctor or pharmacist.

Personal hygiene for men

A build-up of secretions called smegma can form

under the foreskin of uncircumcised men. If you are uncircumcised, gently pull back the foreskin when you have a shower and clean with water. You can use soap if you like, but make sure you rinse it off well.

RELATED SOURCE

https://www.betterhealth.vic.gov.au/health/conditionsandtreatments/personal-hygiene

DESCRIPTION OF THE MACHINE

Lingual-Numeric Calculator

Definition

It is a three-dimensional formula that was designed to complement the work of modern computer in a way that is direct and precise for the advancement of human knowledge. It supports the Pythagorean assertion which says: "All things had their origin and composition in numbers".

It was allegorically expressed as:

First Dimension

Input= [OI x Q] A Slide per Letter

Output In Figures=Cardinal Value

Second Dimension

Input=[1] + [OI x Q] A Slide per Letter

Output In Figures =First Ordinal Value [or the first serial number]

Third Dimension

Input=[OI x P] A Slide per Letter

Output In Figures=Second Ordinal Value [or the second serial number]

Full Meaning Of The Abbreviations:

O-Stands for the overall number of English alphabets [26]

I-Stands for indexes (in descending order) to which the overall number of English alphabets will be multiply by itself. It depends on the number of letters inside a word

Q-Stands for the quantitative value of each letter of English when they are arranged in an alphabetic order

P-Stands for the position of each letter of English when they are arranged in an alphabetic order

For example:

The Quantitative Value Of Each Letter Of English
A=0,B=1,C=2,D=3,E=4,F=5,G=6,H=7,I=8,J=9,K=10,L=11,M=12
N=13,O=14,P=15,Q=16,R=17,S=18,T=19,U=20,V=2

1,W=22,X=23,Y=

Z=25

The Position Of Each Letter Of English

A=1,B=2,C=3,D=4,E=5,F=6,G=7,H=8,I=9,J=10,K=1

1,L=12,M=13N=14,O=15,

P=16,Q=17,R=18,S=19,T=20,U=21,V=22,W=23,X=

24,Y=25,Z=25

Algorithm

-Input

Input can be any word of interest. It can be a name of

disease, term, course, discipline etc

-Data

Data is the representation of `a word in accordance

with the three components of the   machine, namely:

overall number, indexes and quantity

-Computing

Computing is the act of reading a word according to

the computational system of the machine.

-Output

Output are two: in figures and in words:

-Output in figures is the cardinal or ordinal value of

an input.

 -Output in word are vocabularies or sentences

recognized by the

machine during the process of interpretation of an input

Language Of The Machine:

The basic difference between computer and lingual-numeric calculator is the language of the machine: the former understands 0 & 1[mechanically: 'on' & 'off'], while the later understands1 & 1 [literally: 'relevant' or 'irrelevant' based on 'characters']

Mechanism Of Data Processing For An Output

Firstly, upon entering an input, the machine will ask you to select from one of the three dimensions of the formula. Secondly, it will derive an ordinal scale from the obtained value for segmented coding. Thirdly, the machine is going to compute the value obtained into the language of the machine for integrated coding. Fourthly, the machine will start working on various sets of database [e.g. f1, f2, f3, f4, etc] for output processing. It categorizes words into two supporting components, such as: vocabulary [one or more] and sentence [one or more].

Vocabulary- only the relevant words would be recognized by the machine, while the irrelevant words would not be recognized for lack of associated characters literally or metaphorically.

- Sentence- the machine would only recognize a sentence whose integrated code doesn't contradict the integrated code of the subject in a sentence and the general contents of the first component

Segmented Code:

Is the act of considering all the numbers inside the cardinal or ordinal value of an input when making interpretation, it always requires an ordinal scale.

Integrated Code:

Is the act of considering a number reduced into the language of the machine from the cardinal or ordinal value of an input when making interpretation. It can be dependent or independent.

For example-it is dependent when it was used to interpret an ordinal scale of other input, but it is independent when it was used to interpret itself.

Method Of Database Processing Used By The Machine:

F1=[1-letter word database]

F2=[2-letter word database]

F3=[3-letter word database]

F4=[4-letter word database]

F5=[5-letter word database] up to F22=[22-letter word database]

Hence, any word with more than 22 letters would be read as coined word whose morphemes will be computed separately, before joining into one word.

RELATED SOURCE

Rahali lawali: lingual –numeric calculator

www.ingramcontent.com/pod-product-compliance
Lightning Source LLC
Chambersburg PA
CBHW020620220526
45463CB00006B/2632